NIGHT DREAM JOURNAL

Dream Catcher

Copyright © Red Dot, 2019

Disclaimer

All Rights Reserved. No part of this book may be reproduced or transmitted in any form or by any means, mechanical or electronic, including photocopying or recording, or by any information storage and retrieval system, or transmitted by email without permission in writing from the publisher. This book is for entertainment purposes only. The views expressed are those of the author alone.

Dream Journal

Date: _____

Waking Time: _____

Dream Place:

People Met:

What Happened:

Notes:

Dream Journal

Date: _____

Waking Time: _____

Dream Place:

People Met:

What Happened:

Notes:

Dream Journal

Date: _____

Waking Time: _____

Dream Place:

People Met:

What Happened:

Notes:

Dream Journal

Date: _____

Waking Time: _____

Dream Place:

People Met:

What Happened:

Notes:

Dream Journal

Date: _____

Waking Time: _____

Dream Place:

People Met:

What Happened:

Notes:

Dream Journal

Date: _____

Waking Time: _____

Dream Place:

People Met:

What Happened:

Notes:

Dream Journal

Date: _____

Waking Time: _____

Dream Place:

People Met:

What Happened:

Notes:

Dream Journal

Date: _____

Waking Time: _____

Dream Place:

People Met:

What Happened:

Notes:

Dream Journal

Date: _____

Waking Time: _____

Dream Place:

People Met:

What Happened:

Notes:

Dream Journal

Date: _____

Waking Time: _____

Dream Place:

People Met:

What Happened:

Notes:

Dream Journal

Date: _____

Waking Time: _____

Dream Place:

People Met:

What Happened:

Notes:

Dream Journal

Date: _____

Waking Time: _____

Dream Place:

People Met:

What Happened:

Notes:

Dream Journal

Date: _____

Waking Time: _____

Dream Place:

People Met:

What Happened:

Notes:

Dream Journal

Date: _____

Waking Time: _____

Dream Place:

People Met:

What Happened:

Notes:

Dream Journal

Date: _____

Waking Time: _____

Dream Place:

People Met:

What Happened:

Notes:

Dream Journal

Date: _____

Waking Time: _____

Dream Place:

People Met:

What Happened:

Notes:

Dream Journal

Date: _____

Waking Time: _____

Dream Place:

People Met:

What Happened:

Notes:

Dream Journal

Date: _____

Waking Time: _____

Dream Place:

People Met:

What Happened:

Notes:

Dream Journal

Date: _____

Waking Time: _____

Dream Place:

People Met:

What Happened:

Notes:

Dream Journal

Date: _____

Waking Time: _____

Dream Place:

People Met:

What Happened:

Notes:

Dream Journal

Date: _____

Waking Time: _____

Dream Place:

People Met:

What Happened:

Notes:

Dream Journal

Date: _____

Waking Time: _____

Dream Place:

People Met:

What Happened:

Notes:

Dream Journal

Date: _____

Waking Time: _____

Dream Place:

People Met:

What Happened:

Notes:

Dream Journal

Date: _____

Waking Time: _____

Dream Place:

People Met:

What Happened:

Notes:

Dream Journal

Date: _____

Waking Time: _____

Dream Place:

People Met:

What Happened:

Notes:

Dream Journal

Date: _____

Waking Time: _____

Dream Place:

People Met:

What Happened:

Notes:

Dream Journal

Date: _____

Waking Time: _____

Dream Place:

People Met:

What Happened:

Notes:

Dream Journal

Date: _____

Waking Time: _____

Dream Place:

People Met:

What Happened:

Notes:

Dream Journal

Date: _____

Waking Time: _____

Dream Place:

People Met:

What Happened:

Notes:

Dream Journal

Date: _____

Waking Time: _____

Dream Place:

People Met:

What Happened:

Notes:

Dream Journal

Date: _____

Waking Time: _____

Dream Place:

People Met:

What Happened:

Notes:

Dream Journal

Date: _____

Waking Time: _____

Dream Place:

People Met:

What Happened:

Notes:

Dream Journal

Date: _____

Waking Time: _____

Dream Place:

People Met:

What Happened:

Notes:

Dream Journal

Date: _____

Waking Time: _____

Dream Place:

People Met:

What Happened:

Notes:

Dream Journal

Date: _____

Waking Time: _____

Dream Place:

People Met:

What Happened:

Notes:

Dream Journal

Date: _____

Waking Time: _____

Dream Place:

People Met:

What Happened:

Notes:

Dream Journal

Date: _____

Waking Time: _____

Dream Place:

People Met:

What Happened:

Notes:

Dream Journal

Date: _____

Waking Time: _____

Dream Place:

People Met:

What Happened:

Notes:

Dream Journal

Date: _____

Waking Time: _____

Dream Place:

People Met:

What Happened:

Notes:

Dream Journal

Date: _____

Waking Time: _____

Dream Place:

People Met:

What Happened:

Notes:

Dream Journal

Date: _____

Waking Time: _____

Dream Place: People Met:

What Happened:

Notes:

Dream Journal

Date: _____

Waking Time: _____

Dream Place:

People Met:

What Happened:

Notes:

Dream Journal

Date: _____

Waking Time: _____

Dream Place:

People Met:

What Happened:

Notes:

Dream Journal

Date: _____

Waking Time: _____

Dream Place:

People Met:

What Happened:

Notes:

Dream Journal

Date: _____

Waking Time: _____

Dream Place:

People Met:

What Happened:

Notes:

Dream Journal

Date: _____

Waking Time: _____

Dream Place:

People Met:

What Happened:

Notes:

Dream Journal

Date: _____

Waking Time: _____

Dream Place:　　　　　　　People Met:

What Happened:

Notes:

Dream Journal

Date: _____

Waking Time: _____

Dream Place:

People Met:

What Happened:

Notes:

Dream Journal

Date: _____

Waking Time: _____

Dream Place:

People Met:

What Happened:

Notes:

Dream Journal

Date: _____

Waking Time: _____

Dream Place:

People Met:

What Happened:

Notes:

Dream Journal

Date: _____

Waking Time: _____

Dream Place:

People Met:

What Happened:

Notes:

Dream Journal

Date: _____

Waking Time: _____

Dream Place:

People Met:

What Happened:

Notes:

Dream Journal

Date: _____

Waking Time: _____

Dream Place:

People Met:

What Happened:

Notes:

Dream Journal

Date: _____

Waking Time: _____

Dream Place:

People Met:

What Happened:

Notes:

Dream Journal

Date: _____

Waking Time: _____

Dream Place:

People Met:

What Happened:

Notes:

Dream Journal

Date: _____

Waking Time: _____

Dream Place:

People Met:

What Happened:

Notes:

Dream Journal

Date: _____

Waking Time: _____

Dream Place:

People Met:

What Happened:

Notes:

Dream Journal

Date: _____

Waking Time: _____

Dream Place:

People Met:

What Happened:

Notes:

Dream Journal

Date: _____

Waking Time: _____

Dream Place:

People Met:

What Happened:

Notes:

Dream Journal

Date: _____

Waking Time: _____

Dream Place:	People Met:

What Happened:

Notes:

Dream Journal

Date: _____

Waking Time: _____

Dream Place:

People Met:

What Happened:

Notes:

Dream Journal

Date: _____

Waking Time: _____

Dream Place:

People Met:

What Happened:

Notes:

Dream Journal

Date: _____

Waking Time: _____

Dream Place:

People Met:

What Happened:

Notes:

Dream Journal

Date: _____

Waking Time: _____

Dream Place:

People Met:

What Happened:

Notes:

Dream Journal

Date: _____

Waking Time: _____

Dream Place:

People Met:

What Happened:

Notes:

Dream Journal

Date: _____

Waking Time: _____

Dream Place:

People Met:

What Happened:

Notes:

Dream Journal

Date: _____

Waking Time: _____

Dream Place:

People Met:

What Happened:

Notes:

Dream Journal

Date: _____

Waking Time: _____

Dream Place:

People Met:

What Happened:

Notes:

Dream Journal

Date: _____

Waking Time: _____

Dream Place:

People Met:

What Happened:

Notes:

Dream Journal

Date: _____

Waking Time: _____

Dream Place:

People Met:

What Happened:

Notes:

Dream Journal

Date: _____

Waking Time: _____

Dream Place:

People Met:

What Happened:

Notes:

Dream Journal

Date: _____

Waking Time: _____

Dream Place:

People Met:

What Happened:

Notes:

Dream Journal

Date: _____

Waking Time: _____

Dream Place:

People Met:

What Happened:

Notes:

Dream Journal

Date: _____

Waking Time: _____

Dream Place:

People Met:

What Happened:

Notes:

Dream Journal

Date: _____

Waking Time: _____

Dream Place: People Met:

What Happened:

Notes:

Dream Journal

Date: _____

Waking Time: _____

Dream Place:

People Met:

What Happened:

Notes:

Dream Journal

Date: _____

Waking Time: _____

Dream Place:

People Met:

What Happened:

Notes:

Dream Journal

Date: _____

Waking Time: _____

Dream Place: People Met:

What Happened:

Notes:

Dream Journal

Date: _____

Waking Time: _____

Dream Place:

People Met:

What Happened:

Notes:

Dream Journal

Date: _____

Waking Time: _____

Dream Place:

People Met:

What Happened:

Notes:

Dream Journal

Date: _____

Waking Time: _____

Dream Place:

People Met:

What Happened:

Notes:

Dream Journal

Date: _____

Waking Time: _____

Dream Place:

People Met:

What Happened:

Notes:

Dream Journal

Date: _____

Waking Time: _____

Dream Place:

People Met:

What Happened:

Notes:

Dream Journal

Date: _____

Waking Time: _____

Dream Place: People Met:

What Happened:

Notes:

Dream Journal

Date: _____

Waking Time: _____

Dream Place:

People Met:

What Happened:

Notes:

Dream Journal

Date: _____

Waking Time: _____

Dream Place:

People Met:

What Happened:

Notes:

Dream Journal

Date: _____

Waking Time: _____

Dream Place:

People Met:

What Happened:

Notes:

Dream Journal

Date: _____

Waking Time: _____

Dream Place:

People Met:

What Happened:

Notes:

Dream Journal

Date: _____

Waking Time: _____

Dream Place:

People Met:

What Happened:

Notes:

Dream Journal

Date: _____

Waking Time: _____

Dream Place:

People Met:

What Happened:

Notes:

Dream Journal

Date: _____

Waking Time: _____

Dream Place:

People Met:

What Happened:

Notes:

Dream Journal

Date: _____

Waking Time: _____

Dream Place:

People Met:

What Happened:

Notes:

Dream Journal

Date: _____

Waking Time: _____

Dream Place:

People Met:

What Happened:

Notes:

Dream Journal

Date: _____

Waking Time: _____

Dream Place:

People Met:

What Happened:

Notes:

Dream Journal

Date: _____

Waking Time: _____

Dream Place:

People Met:

What Happened:

Notes:

Dream Journal

Date: _____

Waking Time: _____

Dream Place:

People Met:

What Happened:

Notes:

Dream Journal

Date: _____

Waking Time: _____

Dream Place:

People Met:

What Happened:

Notes:

Dream Journal

Date: _____

Waking Time: _____

Dream Place:

People Met:

What Happened:

Notes:

Dream Journal

Date: _____

Waking Time: _____

Dream Place:

People Met:

What Happened:

Notes:

Dream Journal

Date: _____

Waking Time: _____

Dream Place:

People Met:

What Happened:

Notes:

Dream Journal

Date: _____

Waking Time: _____

Dream Place:

People Met:

What Happened:

Notes:

Dream Journal

Date: _____

Waking Time: _____

Dream Place:

People Met:

What Happened:

Notes:

Dream Journal

Date: _____

Waking Time: _____

Dream Place:

People Met:

What Happened:

Notes:

Dream Journal

Date: _____

Waking Time: _____

Dream Place:

People Met:

What Happened:

Notes:

Dream Journal

Date: _____

Waking Time: _____

Dream Place:

People Met:

What Happened:

Notes:

Dream Journal

Date: _____

Waking Time: _____

Dream Place:

People Met:

What Happened:

Notes:

Dream Journal

Date: _____

Waking Time: _____

Dream Place: People Met:

What Happened:

Notes:

Dream Journal

Date: _____

Waking Time: _____

Dream Place:

People Met:

What Happened:

Notes:

Dream Journal

Date: _____

Waking Time: _____

Dream Place:

People Met:

What Happened:

Notes:

Dream Journal

Date: _____

Waking Time: _____

Dream Place:

People Met:

What Happened:

Notes:

Dream Journal

Date: _____

Waking Time: _____

Dream Place:

People Met:

What Happened:

Notes:

Dream Journal

Date: _____

Waking Time: _____

Dream Place:

People Met:

What Happened:

Notes:

Dream Journal

Date: _____

Waking Time: _____

Dream Place:

People Met:

What Happened:

Notes:

Dream Journal

Date: _____

Waking Time: _____

Dream Place:

People Met:

What Happened:

Notes:

Dream Journal

Date: _____

Waking Time: _____

Dream Place:

People Met:

What Happened:

Notes:

Dream Journal

Date: _____

Waking Time: _____

Dream Place:

People Met:

What Happened:

Notes:

Dream Journal

Date: _____

Waking Time: _____

Dream Place:

People Met:

What Happened:

Notes:

Dream Journal

Date: _____

Waking Time: _____

Dream Place:

People Met:

What Happened:

Notes:

Dream Journal

Date: _____

Waking Time: _____

Dream Place:

People Met:

What Happened:

Notes:

Dream Journal

Date: _____

Waking Time: _____

Dream Place:

People Met:

What Happened:

Notes:

Dream Journal

Date: _____

Waking Time: _____

Dream Place:

People Met:

What Happened:

Notes:

Dream Journal

Date: _____

Waking Time: _____

Dream Place:

People Met:

What Happened:

Notes:

Dream Journal

Date: _____

Waking Time: _____

Dream Place:

People Met:

What Happened:

Notes:

Dream Journal

Date: _____

Waking Time: _____

Dream Place:

People Met:

What Happened:

Notes:

Dream Journal

Date: _____

Waking Time: _____

Dream Place:

People Met:

What Happened:

Notes:

Dream Journal

Date: _____

Waking Time: _____

Dream Place:

People Met:

What Happened:

Notes:

Dream Journal

Date: _____

Waking Time: _____

Dream Place:

People Met:

What Happened:

Notes:

Dream Journal

Date: _____

Waking Time: _____

Dream Place:

People Met:

What Happened:

Notes:

Dream Journal

Date: _____

Waking Time: _____

Dream Place:

People Met:

What Happened:

Notes:

Dream Journal

Date: _____

Waking Time: _____

Dream Place:

People Met:

What Happened:

Notes:

Dream Journal

Date: _____

Waking Time: _____

Dream Place: People Met:

What Happened:

Notes:

Dream Journal

Date: _____

Waking Time: _____

Dream Place:

People Met:

What Happened:

Notes:

Made in United States
Orlando, FL
08 November 2022